# Overcoming Nephrotic Syndrome: My Journey to Healing

Andrew young

# DEDICATION

To my mum who always inspired me to speak my truth and let my story be a beacon of light to those searching in the dark.

# CONTENTS

# INTRODUCTION

## A Journey of Triumph and Transformation

In "Overcoming Nephrotic Syndrome: My Journey to Healing," we step into Andrew's world as he opens the doors to his past, sharing his experiences, emotions, and the profound insights he gained throughout his transformative journey. Through the pages of this book, we are invited to witness his struggle with an insidious kidney condition, his quest for answers amidst medical uncertainties, and his unyielding determination to rewrite the narrative of his life. The book begins with a glimpse into Andrew's vibrant life, filled with joy, family, and adventure. Little did he know that his journey would soon take a dramatic turn, introducing him to the bewildering world of nephrotic syndrome. As we journey alongside him, we gain insight into the debilitating symptoms that slowly crept into his life, leading to pain, discomfort, and ultimately, a fateful moment of realisation that pushed him to seek medical intervention.

The initial chapters delve deep into the mysteries of nephrotic syndrome, introducing us to the complex interplay within the body that gave rise to his condition. Andrew's vivid descriptions take us through his physical and emotional struggles, painting a vivid picture of the battles he fought within himself. We witness his determination to understand the root cause of his illness, his frustration in the face of medical ambiguity, and the burden of facing a future that seemed dominated by medications and dialysis.

As the narrative unfolds, a chance encounter in Turkey becomes a turning point – a glimmer of hope that paves the way for Andrew's journey of self-discovery. Fuelled by newfound determination, he dives into research, exploring the intricate connections between his body, energy flow, metaphysics, and the chemistry of the human system. We follow him as he delves into the world of herbs, spirituality, and holistic wellness, slowly but surely transforming from a bystander in his own health to an empowered seeker of answers.

The pivotal moment of revelation arrives when Andrew unravels the link between his emotions and his kidney health. He uncovers how his empathic nature and sensitivity played a role in triggering his condition. This "Eureka moment" becomes a catalyst for profound change as he adopts mindfulness, meditation, and yoga to manage stress and anxiety. Andrew's journey of self-mastery is characterised by a growing understanding of his body's signals and an empowering shift in his relationship with his emotions. The later chapters chronicle Andrew's meticulous steps towards regaining control over his health. We witness his empowered decisions to manage his diet, shed excess weight, and gradually reduce his medication dosage. The steady progress he makes is underscored by his clinic visits transforming from weekly to monthly, then every six months – a reflection of the remarkable healing journey he embarks upon.

Finally, the book concludes with an epilogue that encapsulates Andrew's transformation – physically, emotionally, and spiritually. His narrative transitions from a story of struggle to one of triumph, a testament to the power of understanding, resilience, and the unwavering belief in one's capacity to heal. Andrew's journey is an inspiring reminder that even in the face of seemingly insurmountable odds, the human spirit has the capacity to rise, adapt, and rewrite the story of its own healing.

# CHAPTER 1: UNVEILING THE SILENT STRUGLE

Hello, I'm Andrew. Life was going well for me – spending time with my loved ones, going on vacations, and cherishing every moment. Then, at the age of 22, my journey took an unexpected turn. I was diagnosed with nephrotic syndrome, a condition that affects the kidneys and can disrupt the normal functioning of the body.

Nephrotic syndrome isn't something you can easily spot. It's a silent struggle that goes on inside your body, causing problems without showing obvious signs. The kidneys, those small bean-shaped organs, were my foes in this battle. They started working against each other, sabotaging their own function.

This sneaky condition began with something as simple as constipation. I didn't realise it at the time, but it was a signal that something was amiss in my body. The discomfort grew, and I started experiencing intense stomach pain. It was a pain that wouldn't let go, and I found myself resorting to unusual positions just to get a moment of relief.

As life went on, the pain became a constant companion. I was a driver, often taking long journeys from Leicester to London and back. But my feet would become stiff, almost as if they were rebelling against the road. It became clear that I couldn't keep up with those long journeys anymore. It was frustrating, and I began to wonder why my body was betraying me.

One day, while I was out and about, things took a dramatic

turn. Walking back from shopping, I suddenly felt like the energy was being drained out of me. My breathing became difficult, and my legs seemed to weigh a ton. It was a terrifying experience, one that prompted me to seek medical help immediately. I rushed to Hammersmith Hospital, where my battle against nephrotic syndrome truly began.

Little did I know, that was just the beginning of a journey filled with uncertainties, questions, and discoveries. The doctors ran tests and diagnosed me with nephrotic syndrome. They put me on steroids, various medications, and even discussed the possibility of dialysis – a procedure where a machine would take over some kidney functions. It was overwhelming, to say the least.

My story, though, was far from over. This diagnosis sparked a fire within me, a determination to understand why this was happening to me and how I could overcome it. With each step I took, I discovered more about nephrotic syndrome, the kidneys, and my own body. Join me as I share the chapters of my journey, from the uncertainty of diagnosis to the triumph of finding a way to heal.

# 2 CHAPTER NAME

In medical terms, Nephrotic syndrome is a complex medical condition characterized by a constellation of symptoms arising from kidney dysfunction. It stands as a poignant exemplar of the intricate interplay between the body's physiological systems and the intricate harmony required for homeostasis.

At its core, nephrotic syndrome is a result of perturbations within the glomerular filtration apparatus, the delicate sieving mechanism nestled within the kidney's nephrons. These nephrons, akin to nature's own filtration factories, are responsible for sifting through the blood, removing waste products, and maintaining the delicate balance of fluids and electrolytes.

In the case of nephrotic syndrome, this precise filtration process is jeopardised, leading to the leakage of essential proteins, such as albumin, from the blood into the urine. This leakage, aptly termed proteinuria, ensues a cascade of effects that engenders the classical hallmarks of the syndrome.

The intricate dance between oncotic and hydrostatic pressures becomes disrupted, triggering a decrease in serum albumin levels. This drop in albumin precipitates a decrease in plasma oncotic pressure, resulting in a state of hypoproteinaemia. The body, in its tireless attempt to restore equilibrium, responds by promoting sodium and water retention, which exacerbates oedema—particularly in dependent areas like the ankles and periorbital regions. This clinical manifestation of oedema is an unmistakable emblem of the nephrotic syndrome.

Furthermore, the decrease in albumin levels prompts the liver to ramp up its synthesis of lipoproteins, as albumin is pivotal for lipid transport. This elevated synthesis culminates in hyperlipidaemia, characteristically showcasing as elevated levels of cholesterol and triglycerides in the blood. The shimmering

lipid-rich serum becomes a visual testament to the intricate web of physiological responses elicited by the syndrome.

The underlying aetiology of nephrotic syndrome is diverse, ranging from primary glomerular pathologies like minimal change disease to secondary causes such as diabetes mellitus and systemic lupus erythematosus. The immune system's role in certain cases underscores the intricate labyrinth of immunological crossroads that can culminate in renal pathology.

This perplexing syndrome began its invasion in a seemingly innocent way – with constipation and at times, suffering with swollen feet. But beneath this seemingly unrelated issue, something much more intricate was at play. As the days went by, the discomfort escalated, eventually manifesting as severe stomach pain. The pain was unlike anything I had experienced before, so intense that I had to contort myself into strange positions just to catch a brief moment of relief.

Imagine trying to live your life while being constantly besieged by this pain. It's like an invisible enemy, sapping your energy and clouding your days. The situation was made even more complex by my history as a driver. Those long journeys between Leicester and London, once routine, became tests of endurance. The pain in my stomach wasn't the only problem – my feet would stiffen and seize up, making it clear that something was seriously amiss.

**Overcoming Nephrotic Syndrome: My Journey to Healing**

It's a strange sensation, realising that your body, which you've always relied on, can suddenly turn against you. That's what nephrotic syndrome did – it turned my own kidneys, those vital components that help keep my body healthy, into adversaries. And so, the mystery deepened as I sought answers, determined to understand why this was happening and how I could reclaim control over my body. The journey to unravel these mysteries was just beginning, and little did I know that it would lead me to revelations that would transform my understanding of health and healing.

# 3 CHAPTER NAME

There are moments in life that act as turning points, steering us in unforeseen directions. For me, one of those moments occurred during a seemingly ordinary shopping trip. As I walked, I felt an inexplicable sensation – it was as if life itself was slowly seeping out of me. Each step became a struggle, and even the act of breathing felt more laborious than it should be. This was a stark departure from the vibrant life I had known, and it was clear that something was seriously amiss.

In response to this alarming experience, my instincts kicked in, and I made a beeline for the hospital. The journey from that shopping trip to the hospital marked a transition from confusion to determination, from uncertainty to seeking answers.

The hospital became a place of tests, consultations, and exploration. The medical professionals diligently worked to uncover the truth behind my mysterious symptoms. Those days turned into weeks, and weeks into two whole months – a period where my life felt like it was on pause.

Finally, the pieces of the puzzle started coming together. The diagnosis was revealed: nephrotic syndrome. This marked a pivotal moment in my journey, a moment where the unknown transformed into clarity, though accompanied by a mixture of emotions – relief for finally having a name for my ailment and apprehension for the road that lay ahead.

Treatment plans were put into motion. My daily routine underwent a seismic shift as steroids, blood thinners, and a slew of tablets became my constant companions. Life took on a new rhythm, with medications dictating my schedule and hospital visits becoming a regular occurrence.

The familiar comfort of my previous routines was replaced by an unfamiliar landscape of medical terms, prescriptions, and therapeutic interventions. It was as if my body had become a battleground for a fight that I hadn't signed up for.

Yet, even in the midst of this upheaval, a flicker of determination ignited within me. The turning point wasn't just a moment of diagnosis; it was also the birth of a resolve to confront this challenge head-on, to understand it, and ultimately, to conquer it. The road ahead was unclear, but my spirit was unwavering. With each passing day, I was inching closer to not only overcoming nephrotic syndrome but also discovering the strength within myself that I never knew existed.

# 4 CHAPTER NAME

Leaving the hospital after a prolonged stay marked a definitive transition into a new phase of my ongoing battle against nephrotic syndrome. The resounding clang of the hospital doors closing behind me seemed to encapsulate both liberation and trepidation, as I ventured into the world outside with a sense of both relief and apprehension. Although physically separated from a journey of spending time as an inpatient on a critical ward with bustling medical staff, the weight of my condition lingered persistently, akin to an uninvited guest overstaying its welcome.

My routine now revolved around a cycles of clinic visits. With the regularity of clockwork, I found myself returning each week to the familiar realm of the hospital. The waiting rooms, often bustling with patients bearing their own health burdens, became a zone of shared experiences and silent empathy. The mere presence of others going through their own struggles provided a peculiar yet comforting camaraderie, as we all navigated the complexities of our respective journeys. Amid these visits, the doctors and specialists took on the role of my navigational guides, steering me through the intricate labyrinth of medical decisions and therapeutic choices.

Yet, even within the encompassing embrace of those sterile walls, comprehensive answers remained elusive, and a shroud of uncertainty cloaked my days. Conversations with the medical experts, while illuminating in some aspects, often led to corridors of ambiguity. They likened nephrotic syndrome to an internal battleground, a ceaseless clash where my own kidneys were protagonists entangled in an unrelenting struggle. Yet, when I yearned for information about the origins of this internecine conflict, the responses were frustratingly nebulous. This shared frustration seemed to bind me with the fellow occupants of the waiting room—a silent fraternity born of the shared pursuit of understanding the enigma afflicting us.

The notion that this syndrome was destined to be my lifelong companion felt like an unwieldy load upon my shoulders. Contemplating a future characterized by medications, potential dialysis sessions, and perpetual dependency painted an intimidating portrait of the path ahead. The very idea suffocated me at times, as if I were trapped in an unending cycle of illness and reliance. The life that was once my own, marked by vigor and autonomy, appeared to slip further into the recesses of memory with each passing day. In its place emerged the somber tableau of a future seemingly preordained by my diagnosis, a landscape fraught with both challenges and an unflagging determination to confront them.

# 5 CHAPTER NAME

In Turkey, amidst the vibrant energy of a foreign land, I crossed paths with a woman who had been living with nephrotic syndrome for a staggering 15 years. She was a testament to resilience, living her life despite the challenges – dialysis and all. Her mere existence became a glimmer of hope in the midst of my own struggles. It was as if her experience shattered the bleak clouds that had been gathering around me, allowing a ray of light to filter through.

In a profound way, her story acted as a catalyst for a profound transformation within me. It served as a piercing wake-up call, a reverberating reminder that while the battle I was fighting was undoubtedly arduous, it was by no means insurmountable. Infused with this newfound wellspring of hope, I embarked on an exhilarating expedition of research and self-discovery, propelled by an insatiable thirst to unveil the hidden dimensions of my own capabilities.

The sacrifices of time and effort I made were, without a doubt, a small price to pay for the wealth of knowledge and insight I harvested. This expedition transcended the realm of medical inquiry and became an expedition of personal growth, a metamorphic journey that reshaped me from a mere combatant of a health condition into an avid pupil of existence itself. Armed with a growing treasury of comprehension, I felt determined to recalibrate the trajectory of my journey. The glimmer of hope that had first ignited during that serendipitous encounter in Turkey had now swelled into a roaring blaze. Its radiant light illuminated the path ahead, imbuing me with the vigor to confront and conquer the formidable challenges that awaited me.

Even as the composition of my social circle may have shifted, the knowledge I had accrued proved to be an enduring treasure. Bolstered by this newfound understanding, I became resolute in my mission to turn the tides of fortune in my favor. The flicker of hope ignited by that chance encounter had evolved into an unwavering conflagration, providing both illumination and warmth as I forged ahead, invigorated by the strength to navigate the labyrinthine twists of my narrative.

# 6 CHAPTER NAME

Life is a puzzle, and sometimes, the pieces fall into place when we least expect it. As I delved deeper into my studies, seeking to unravel the mysteries of my nephrotic syndrome, I stumbled upon a revelation that would change everything. It was a eureka moment that unveiled the intricate connection between my kidney issue and the emotions that coursed through me.

It was like finding the missing piece of a jigsaw puzzle. My extensive research had led me to a realisation: my kidney troubles were intrinsically tied to stress and emotional turmoil. I was not just a passive observer of my own feelings; I was an empath, someone who felt the emotions of others deeply. This sensitivity had unwittingly become a key player in the battle within my body.

When I became upset, anxious, or overwhelmed, my kidneys bore the brunt of my emotional turbulence. The very adrenaline that should have been aiding me in fight or flight situations took an unexpected detour into my kidneys. It was a baffling phenomenon, a reaction born from the intricate interplay between the mind and the body.

I hungered for knowledge, craving a deeper understanding of the intricate workings of the body. The kidneys, those enigmatic filters, held secrets that I was determined to uncover. I delved into topics as diverse as energy flow, metaphysics, and the chemistry of the body. My thirst for knowledge transformed me into what some might call a "study nerd." I pored over books, articles, and resources, seeking answers that had thus far eluded me.

# Overcoming Nephrotic Syndrome: My Journey to Healing

This journey of discovery came at a price. As I delved deeper into my studies, I began to drift away from some friends. The conversations that once filled our interactions seemed shallow and insignificant compared to the revelations I was uncovering. My focus had shifted, and it was a lonely path at times. However, the friends who remained were the ones who recognised the fire within me, the burning desire to understand and overcome this condition that had disrupted my life.

Imagine the scenario: an everyday situation causes stress or discomfort, triggering a surge of adrenaline – the body's natural response to stress. But for me, as an empath, this energy surge had nowhere to go. I wasn't facing a physical threat that required me to fight or flee. Instead, this excess adrenaline found its way into my kidneys, unleashing a cascade of physiological reactions that wreaked havoc on my body.

It was a revelation that explained so much. The excruciating pain, the fluctuations in my condition – all could be traced back to this hidden connection. It was as if my body was trying to process emotions and responses in a way that had unintended consequences for my kidneys.

This newfound understanding wasn't just a scientific revelation; it was a revelation about myself. I had unknowingly been carrying the weight of not only my own emotions but also the emotions of those around me. This sensitivity, while a gift in many ways, had inadvertently become a source of distress for my own body.

As I connected the dots, a renewed sense of purpose filled me. I wasn't just dealing with a medical condition; I was uncovering the layers of my own being. Armed with this knowledge, I was determined to find a way to harness my emotions, to navigate stress and anxiety in a way that wouldn't compromise my health. The eureka moment had ignited a fire within me, a determination to not only understand but to transform the course of my journey towards healing.

# 7 CHAPTER NAME

Armed with the knowledge of the intricate connection between my emotions and my kidney health, I embarked on a new chapter of my journey – a chapter marked by empowerment, self-discovery, and the reclamation of control over my body and mind.

The first step in this transformation was embracing mindfulness, yoga, and meditation. These practices became my allies in taming the emotional roller coaster that had inadvertently triggered my kidney issues. Mindfulness, the art of being present in the moment, allowed me to observe my emotions without becoming entangled in them. Yoga and meditation, with their focus on breath and self-awareness, became tools to manage stress and anxiety.

But that was just the beginning. I realised that my body needed more than just emotional management. My diet played a pivotal role in my overall well-being. So, armed with a newfound determination, I took charge of what I ate. I sought out foods that nourished my body, foods that were kind to my kidneys. As a result, I started shedding excess weight, a move that had a positive impact on my condition.

The transformation was slow but steady. I could feel the change within me, not just physically but mentally as well. My mind was becoming a calmer place, a sanctuary free from the constant turmoil that had once plagued me. And, as if in response to this newfound harmony, my kidney function began to improve.

The improvement wasn't a sudden miracle, but a gradual process. The pain that had been a constant companion no longer existed. The fluctuations that had been a hallmark of my journey became less erratic. I was reclaiming control over my body, inch by inch, breath by breath.

This progress allowed me to take a bold step. With consultation from my medical team, I made the decision to reduce my medication dosage. It was a leap of faith, a move that reflected my growing confidence in the path I was forging. The medications had been a lifeline, but now, armed with knowledge and mindful practices, I felt ready to take on a new challenge – a life with fewer pills and a stronger focus on holistic well-being.

As I looked back on the journey that had brought me to this point, I marvelled at the transformations that had taken place – both within me and around me. It was more than just overcoming a medical condition; it was a journey of self-discovery, empowerment, and healing. And while the path ahead remained uncertain, one thing was clear – I had taken back the reins of my life, steering it towards a future defined by strength, resilience, and the unwavering belief in the power of the human spirit.

# 8 CHAPTER NAME

The journey of overcoming nephrotic syndrome had become a testament to the resilience of the human spirit. As the pages of my life story turned, I found myself moving from one chapter of struggle to another of triumph. Chapter 8 was titled "Steady Progress," a chapter that highlighted the remarkable strides I had taken in reclaiming my health and my life.

My relationship with the hospital began to change. The once-frequent clinic visits, a constant reminder of my condition, began to space out. From the weekly routine, they shifted to monthly appointments, and eventually, I found myself facing the hospital corridors every six months. Each visit was marked by hopeful anticipation, as I eagerly awaited the results that would reflect the journey I had embarked upon.

The doctors who had walked beside me through the darkest days of my journey were now witnesses to the transformation that was unfolding. Their amazement was palpable as they reviewed my progress. The gradual improvement in my kidney function, the diminishing presence of the symptoms that had once plagued me, all painted a picture of healing that defied conventional expectations.

Reclaiming control over my life wasn't just a metaphor – it was a lived reality. No longer was I solely defined by my diagnosis or tethered to medications. The power of knowledge, self-discovery, and mindful practices had allowed me to rewrite the narrative of my life. The pain and uncertainty that had once shrouded my existence were giving way to hope and possibility.

The journey wasn't just about physical healing; it was a profound journey of self-discovery. With each step I took towards understanding the intricate relationship between my emotions and my health, I unravelled layers of my own identity. I had emerged not just as a survivor but as a student of life, constantly learning and evolving.

As the pages of this chapter turned, the narrative was one of growth and transformation. The journey wasn't linear; there were setbacks and challenges along the way. But each setback became a stepping stone, propelling me forward with renewed determination. This was a chapter marked by progress – steady, relentless progress that affirmed the resilience of the human spirit.

Looking back, I marvelled at the path I had travelled. From the moment of diagnosis to the triumphs of today, it was a journey that encompassed the full spectrum of human experience – pain, uncertainty, hope, and healing. As I turned the pages, I knew that this chapter was just one part of the larger story – a story that would continue to unfold with each new day, each new triumph, and each new moment of growth.

# 9 CHAPTER NAME

As my journey to healing progressed, life continued to weave unexpected encounters into my narrative. In the waiting room of the clinic, on a day when I was well on my way to recovery, I found myself face to face with a figure from my past – an old school friend. This chance meeting would open a new chapter in my understanding of nephrotic syndrome and the varied paths it carved through lives.

As we exchanged greetings, I sensed a mix of surprise and excitement in his demeanour. My friend, like me, had been battling the very same condition. We settled into conversation, reminiscing about school days and eventually delving into the complexities of our shared illness.

Curiosity sparked his questions about my experiences. I detailed the symptoms that had once plagued me – the constipation that led to stomach pain, the breathlessness that clouded my every step. His eagerness grew as he listened, and it wasn't long before he eagerly began drawing parallels between my symptoms and his own.

As he shared his journey, it became clear that his struggles extended beyond the medical realm. His interactions with the clinic staff, the impatience he exhibited in the waiting room, and the short fuse he displayed – all painted a picture of heightened anxiety and stress. It was a vivid reminder that the impacts of an illness often extended far beyond the physical realm, intertwining with emotional and psychological states.

uncertainties, and life events that seemed to bear down heavily. His story resonated with me, a reminder of how external factors could manifest within our bodies, influencing our well-being in unexpected ways.

In that moment, I felt compelled to share the insights I had gathered on my journey. I spoke of the connection between stress, emotions, and the manifestations of nephrotic syndrome. Yet, my words were met with laughter, a dismissal of my findings, and a declaration that even medical professionals were uncertain about the condition's origins and cures.

With a calm resolve, I shared my own story of recovery, of stepping away from medication, and the belief that healing was possible. I explained how I had integrated mindfulness, meditation, and lifestyle changes into my routine, resulting in significant improvements. But his scepticism persisted, his laughter echoing as he went to have his blood tests done.

Little did I know, that conversation would be the closing chapter of my clinic visits. As I walked away from that encounter, I carried not only the memory of our meeting but also a newfound understanding – the journeys of those who share an illness can diverge wildly. Our reactions, beliefs, and paths to healing can be as diverse as the shades of human experience.

As I ventured forward, leaving behind the waiting room and the clinic's sterile walls, I held onto the awareness that while the journey to healing was deeply personal, the connections we formed along the way added layers of complexity and shared resilience to the narrative. It was yet another reminder that our stories, though unique, often intersect with the stories of others, creating a rich tapestry of human experience.

# EPILOGUE: A NEW BEGINNING

As the final chapter of my journey approached, I marvelled at the distance I had travelled. What began as a bewildering diagnosis had evolved into a narrative of triumph, resilience, and self-discovery. The epilogue, titled "A New Beginning," was a reflection of the transformation that had taken place.

Today, I stand not only healthier but stronger than ever before. My journey through the challenges of nephrotic syndrome gifted me with profound insights. I had learned to decipher the language of my body, to embrace mindfulness as a way of life, and to approach wellness holistically. The fear that once clouded my existence had dissipated, replaced by a profound sense of purpose and gratitude.

The epilogue is not just an end; it's a beginning. It's a chapter of life that opens to new possibilities, a canvas waiting to be painted with experiences that celebrate health, joy, and vitality. As I close this chapter, I'm filled with a deep appreciation for the lessons learned, the resilience gained, and the unwavering belief that with determination and understanding, we can rewrite the stories of our lives.

THANK YOU FOR READING